Copyright © 2020 by Amos Jacobs

R.D.N

Table of Contents

INTRODUCTION TO ADRENAL FATIGUE

Adrenal fatigue occurs as a result of chronic stress and adrenal insufficiency. Your adrenal glands are responsible for producing cortisol. Cortisol is a hormone that helps regulate your blood pressure.

When you're stressed, your adrenal glands release cortisol. The cortisol responds to a slowed-down immune system and a change in blood pressure.

When you experience chronic stress or anxiety, your adrenal glands may not produce enough cortisol. This is called adrenal insufficiency, which can be medically diagnosed.

Adrenal fatigue isn't recognized as a medical diagnosis. Only some doctors believe chronic stress and adrenal insufficiency cause adrenal fatigue.

Common Adrenal Fatigue Symptoms

Frustratingly, the symptoms associated with adrenal fatigue are often described by medical professionals as "non-specific," "vague," and "ambiguous."

Many of the symptoms associated with adrenal fatigue could be associated with a number of other syndromes and diseases such as thyroid dysfunction, an autoimmune condition, anxiety, depression, or infection.

These symptoms include:

- Generalized fatigue

- Trouble sleeping or insomnia

- Brain fog and lack of focus and motivation

- Thinning hair and nail discoloration

- Menstrual irregularity

- Low exercise tolerance and recovery

- Low motivation

- Low sex drive

- Cravings, poor appetite, and digestive issues

- Low Blood Pressure

That list may be long, but it's far from complete. Because all your hormones are interconnected, if your cortisol levels are out of whack, your other hormone levels like progesterone, estrogen, and testosterone levels likely will be thrown off too. Meaning that anyone with adrenal fatigue can begin to suffer from other hormonal conditions, which can compound the symptoms and confuse doctors.

Adrenal fatigue is also associated with adrenal insufficiency. Symptoms of adrenal insufficiency include:

- chronic fatigue
- loss of appetite

- stomach pain

- muscle weakness

- unexplained weight loss

WHAT IS THE ADRENAL FATIGUE DIET?

The adrenal fatigue diet is a food-based approach to improving stress on the adrenal glands. Your adrenal glands are located around your kidneys. They produce hormones that help regulate your body.

Adrenal fatigue occurs when your adrenal glands can't function properly.

The adrenal glands sit atop the kidneys and function as exocrine glands that produce a variety of essential-to-life hormones including adrenaline, aldosterone, and cortisol. In short, these hormones are responsible for regulating the body's metabolism, immune system suppression, regulation of blood pressure and electrolyte balance, and the rapid response to stress. After long periods of extreme stress or dysfunction of the adrenal glands (such as with certain diseases or the presence of tumors, etc.) there may be an imbalance of one or more of those hormones either from over- or under-production. To confirm the imbalance or inadequate levels of the adrenal hormones, blood tests are needed. But those common symptoms are also a good indicator that something is wrong.

Lifestyle and diet changes are usually necessary to recover from adrenal fatigue.

HOW TO RECOVER FROM ADRENAL FATIGUE

The common protocol for treating adrenal fatigue is as follows:

i. follow an adrenal fatigue diet which entails avoiding foods that cause inflammation and loading up on anti-inflammatory foods.

ii. eat high-protein foods along with plenty of vegetables and whole grains

iii. avoid refined sugars and processed foods

iv. go to bed early (here's my sleep tips)

v.   take a supplement with B5, B6, and B12 vitamins (under doctor supervision)

vi.   consume foods high in omega-3 fatty acids, curcumin (turmeric), and vitamin C

vii. add adaptogenic herbs to your diet – cordyceps, ashwagandha, rehmannia, and licorice root

viii. hydrate properly throughout the day

ix.   replace any missing nutrients (confirmed by doctor's blood test and under supervision) such as vitamin D, magnesium, zinc, and selenium

x.   rest during the day, as needed

xi.   participate in regular meditation and use other stress-relieving breathing techniques

xii.   do yoga or another mild exercise (as not to create more fatigue)

Our glands may be tiny, but they have powerful abilities to affect how we feel each day and how we manage what comes our way in life. You may have heard of the terms, "adrenal burn-out" or "adrenal fatigue" which mean that the glands have been exhausted beyond their daily duties.

A diet high in stress-inducing chemicals, sugars and certain other properties directly affect your glands. They can disrupt your sleep, hormone function, and your weight and mood.

When you are not feeling your best, the food choices you make become even more important to your health. Especially when your adrenals respond to stress your cell metabolism speeds up, burning many more nutrients normally needed. With adrenal fatigue, the cells have used up much of the body's stored nutrients, creating a nutritional void. Good healthy food is the best source for replenishing these nutrients.

So something you can do right now to improve your diet and support your adrenals is start adding in 'Adrenal Compliant Diet'.

If you are suffering from fatigue, when you eat is very important. By eating healthy food at frequent and regular intervals. This can help avoid low blood sugar and make a difference in your health and energy levels.

Adrenal Fatigue Diet Tips

Breakfast

Breakfast is a highly valuable meal to the body. It is the first time the body gets a taste of energy and all of the nutrients to go with it in over 12 hours {because you're practicing intermittent fasting, right}. Breakfast literally means breaking-the-fast.

Not to mention it is generally the time in which your body is waking up and changing over hormonal flow from nighttime to daytime. Through this transition, your body is running at high-efficiency and is ready to take in what was lost throughout the sleeping hours by replenishing and restoring your body's stores as well as foster the need throughout the day.

Basically, breakfast is a legit meal you shouldn't skip.

Eat breakfast within 1 hour of waking – don't leave it too long to get your cortisol levels into gear.

Don't skip meals especially breakfast – you need to get your blood sugars up at the beginning of the day.

Don't wait too long to eat meals with adrenal fatigue, the body has a difficult time storing energy, to eat smaller meals at regular intervals.

Foods to avoid

If you decide to try an adrenal-friendly diet, doctors recommend limiting foods and drinks high in refined and processed sugar and unhealthy fats, while also managing blood sugar.

Some foods to avoid include:

i.   white sugar

ii.   white flour

iii. alcohol

iv.   caffeine

v.   soda

vi.   fried food

vii. processed food

viii. fast food

ix.   artificial sweeteners

Timing your meals is also important. It helps with regulating blood sugar and supporting adrenal glands.

It helps to eat breakfast, and eat regularly throughout the day. Skipping breakfast and lunch forces your body to burn stored nutrients and reduces your energy levels.

If you eat regular, balanced meals and healthy snacks, you can maintain your energy and cortisol levels all day.

Foods to eat

A well-balanced diet is the best way to keep your body healthy and to regulate your sugar levels. Doctors recommend balancing protein, healthy fats, and high-quality, nutrient-dense carbohydrates.

Increase your vegetable intake to get the necessary amount of vitamins and minerals. Also, include foods high in vitamin C, B vitamins (especially B-5 and B-6), and magnesium to help support healthy adrenal glands.

Some foods to eat on the adrenal fatigue diet include:

- lean meats

- fish

- eggs

- legumes

- nuts

- leafy greens and colorful vegetables

- whole grains

- dairy

- low-sugar fruits

- sea salt in moderation

- healthy fats such as olive oil, coconut oil, and grapeseed oil

It's also important to remain hydrated. Dehydration can influence your stress levels and force your adrenal glands to produce cortisol.

All of us struggle with anxiety from time to time. But when stressful days turn into weeks, and those weeks turn into worn-out months, you may wonder if what you're actually experiencing is adrenal fatigue.

The theory behind the hotly debated condition goes something like this: When your body is in a state of constant, chronic stress, your adrenal glands become less effective at producing cortisol, the stress hormone that has multiple functions, from regulating blood pressure to decreasing inflammation.

It's important to note that this condition is not officially recognized by the majority of conventional medical practitioners, who point to a lack of scientific evidence to support the diagnosis. Many are also concerned that attempts to treat the unproven condition may prevent individuals from properly addressing a deeper underlying health issue.

If you're concerned about any of the symptoms we mentioned earlier and/or are considering taking medications or supplements to address them, step one would be to talk to a health professional.

But regardless of whether you believe in adrenal fatigue, you can start feeling better by simply eating the right foods. Focus on incorporating more whole, real ingredients and cutting out the extra salt and added sugars.

This book contains over twenty recipes with Smoothies and soup that are chock-full of gut-healthy probiotics, lean proteins, healthy fats, and whole grains, all of which can help take you from exhausted to energized and restore the proper function of the adrenal glands.

ADRENAL DIET RECIPES

The adrenal fatigue diet promotes:

i.   proper functionality of the adrenal glands

ii.   healthy blood pressure

iii. increased healthy nutrients in the body

iv.   improved stress levels

This diet is similar to most recommended balanced diets, which generally include:

- high-protein foods

- vegetables

- whole grains

The goal is to increase your energy levels naturally so you don't burn stored nutrients.

1. 10 minute Breakfast Hash with Plantains + Chimichurri

Despite all the attention low carb diets get, resistant starches, like plantains that lower blood sugar and balance insulin, are actually key for adrenal health. Enjoy them in this hash, where, paired with sausage and topped with a zesty herb sauce, they won't taste any different from regular potatoes.

PREP TIME: 5 MINS | COOK TIME: 10 MINS

Serves: 4

INGREDIENTS

Hash

- 1 lb breakfast sausage

- 3 plantains

- 4 Tbsp coconut oil

Chimichurri

- Chimichurri

- ¼ cup red wine vinegar

- ¼ cup balsamic vinegar

- 2 cloves garlic, minced

- 1 shallot, chopped

- 1 jalapeno chili, seeded + Chopped

- ½ cup fresh basil (Thai basil)

- ¼ cup fresh cilantro

- ½ cup olive oil

- 1 tsp salt

Toppings

- 8 eggs {optional}

- Fresh cilantro {optional}

INSTRUCTIONS

Hash

1. Peel and dice the plantains.

2. In a large skillet, brown sausage. Drain and set aside.

3. Add coconut oil to same skillet and heat over medium heat.

4. Once sizzling add diced plantains and let cook, turning to brown each side.

5. Remove plantains once cooked and add to sausage. Mix together and add cilantro if using.

6. Cook eggs as desired {fried, soft, scrambled, etc}

Chimichurri

1. To make chimichurri add red wine vinegar, balsamic, garlic, shallot, jalapeno, basil, cilantro and salt to food processor or blender. Slowly add in olive oil while blending. Set aside to allow flavors to blend.

2. Top plantain and sausage mixture with eggs and drizzle with chimichurri.

2. Healthy, Easy Vegan Chickpea Scramble (Perfect for breakfast)

This chickpea scramble breakfast bowl is my vegan answer to scrambled eggs. Chickpeas are such a interesting ingredient, the water in which the chickpeas sit in their can – known as aquafaba – has amazing, egg-like properties, and can be used for baking or even to make meringues. In this recipe, the aquafaba lends the chickpeas their scrambled egg-like texture.

Prep Time: 10 minutes | Cook Time: 10 minutes

Servings: 2 Bowls

Ingredients

Chickpea Scramble

- 1 15 oz Can of Chickpeas
- 1/2 Tsp Turmeric
- 1/2 Tsp Salt
- 1/2 Tsp Pepper
- 1/4 White Onion diced

- 2 Cloves Garlic minced

- Drizzle Extra Virgin Olive Oil

Breakfast Bowl

- Mixed Greens

- Handful of Parsley minced

- Handful of Cilantro minced

- Avocado

Instructions

Chickpea Scramble

1. In a bowl, pour out chickpeas AND a little bit of the water they're in. Mash chickpeas slightly with a fork, leaving some whole. Mix in turmeric, salt, and pepper until evenly combined.

2. Then, mince garlic and dice onion. Heat a pan over medium heat with a drizzle of olive oil. First, sauté the onions until they are soft. Then add the garlic and continue sautéing until garlic is fragrant - about a minute or so. Be careful not to let garlic brown!

3. When onions and garlic are done, add in mashed chickpeas and sauté for about five minutes.

Breakfast Bowls

1. Assemble the breakfast bowls. Add in some mixed greens at the bottom of the bowls, topped with the chickpea scramble.

2. Top with minced cilantro and parsley. Serve with avocado slices.

Recipe Notes

i.   This bowl would also be delicious topped with coconut bacon.

ii.   Also please note that this recipe is very turmeric-forward. If turmeric's not your thing, feel free to use less or omit altogether.

iii.   Quality protein is a must when you're trying to get your adrenal health under control; while the usual go-tos like fish, eggs, and are no-no's for vegans, never underestimate the power of beans. Here, chickpeas and fresh herbs make for quick and flavorful plant-based breakfast. The pinch of turmeric not only adds some extra anti-inflammatory power but also brightens up the entire bowl.

3. Apple Pecan Quinoa Breakfast

Shredded apples and coconut sugar give this high-fiber breakfast quinoa the perfect touch of sweetness, while pecans provide that essential healthy fat to keep you energized through the morning. It doesn't hurt that the recipe tastes like pie too.

This healthy breakfast recipe is easy enough for every day but tasty enough for company. It may be made ahead and reheated in the oven or stove prior to serving.

Prep Time: 10 mins | Cook Time: 35 mins

Servings: 4

Ingredients

- 4 apples divided

- 1 cup quinoa rinsed

- 1 ¼ cup almond milk or milk of choice

- ¼ cup applesauce

- 3 tablespoons coconut palm sugar

- 1 teaspoon ground cinnamon

- ½ teaspoon sea salt

- 1 teaspoon vanilla extract

- ¼ cup chopped pecans

Optional: Maple syrup for drizzling

Instructions

1. Using a box grater or food processor, shred two apples.

2. Bring quinoa and milk to a simmer in a medium saucepan, stirring often. Stir in grated apples, applesauce, sugar, vanilla, cinnamon and salt. Return to a simmer. Cover and cook on low for 25 minutes.

3. Chop remaining 2 apples. Stir in chopped apples and vanilla and re-cover. Cook for 5 to 10 more minutes. Remove from heat and let sit covered for 5 more minutes.

4. Divide among four serving bowls and top each with a tablespoon of pecans. If desired, drizzle with maple syrup. Serve warm. May

be made ahead and reheated prior to serving.

4. VEGAN CACIO E PEPE WITH GARLICKY MUSHROOMS

You only need a few pantry staples to make this plant-based Cacio e Pepe. Spaghetti gets tossed in a peppery, cheesy sauce and then topped with mushrooms.

Prep Time: 5 Minutes | Cook Time: 25 Minutes

Yield: Serves 4

Ingredients

- 8 ounces spaghetti (gluten-free or regular)

- salt, to taste

- 4 tablespoons of dairy-free butter, divided

- 8 ounces Chanterelle, Oyster, or Cremini mushrooms, roughly chopped

- 3 cloves of garlic, thinly sliced

- 1 teaspoon coarsely ground black pepper, plus more to taste

- 2 ounces vegan parmesan cheese, finely grated

INSTRUCTIONS

1. Cook the Pasta: bring a large pot of salted water to a boil over high heat. Once boiling,

add the pasta and cook until just before al dente – the pasta will finish cooking later.

2. Reserve 1½ cups of starchy water, then drain the pasta and set aside.

3. Sauté the Mushrooms: In the meantime, melt 1 tablespoon of butter in a sauté pan over medium-high heat. Then, add the chopped mushrooms and sauté for 3 to 5 minutes. Add the sliced garlic to the pan and cook for an additional 1 to 2 minutes, until fragrant and translucent.

4. Remove the mushrooms and garlic from the pan and set aside, returning the pan to the burner.

5. Bloom the Pepper: melt 2 tablespoons of butter in the same pan over medium-high heat. Add the freshly ground black pepper and swirl it around in the pan for about a minute to bloom the spice. Then, add ¾ cup of the reserved pasta water to the pan and bring it to a simmer.

6. Add the Pasta: Reduce the heat to low, then add in the pasta and remaining 1 tablespoon of butter. Once the butter has melted, add in the grated parmesan and toss the pasta with tongs, until the dairy-free cheese has melted. If your sauce is too thick, add more pasta water in 2 tablespoon increments to thin it out.

7. Serve: transfer the pasta to serving plates, and top with our caramelized garlicky mushrooms, or as desired. Serve warm; this recipe is best served fresh, but leftovers will keep in the fridge for up to 3 days and are best reheated on the stovetop with a splash of water.

5. Fluffy Sweet Potato Breakfast Bowls

These Sweet Potato Breakfast Bowls are a healthy and hearty way to enjoy your morning meal. They're also Vegan, Gluten Free, Sugar Free and Grain Free.

These sweet little spuds have made their way onto our lunch and dinner plates, so why is it that we don't enjoy them for breakfast as well. The combination of pomegranate, pumpkin seeds, cacao nibs, coconut yogurt, and some Easy Vegan Granola is very, very refreshing.

Prep Time: 10 minutes | Cook Time: 45 minutes

Yield: Serves 2

INGREDIENTS

- 2 medium sweet potatoes
- 2/3 cup non-dairy milk
- 2 tablespoons ground flax
- 1 tablespoon nut or seed butter of choice (I used cashew)

- 2 teaspoons vanilla extract

- 1 teaspoon cinnamon

- Pinch of salt

Optional Toppings: pomegranate, pumpkin seeds, coconut yogurt, cacao nibs, and/or granola

INSTRUCTIONS

1. Preheat your oven to 400F and line a baking tray with parchment paper or a silicone mat. Wash the sweet potatoes, but do not peel them. Piece the potatoes a few times with a knife, then place on the tray and bake for 45 to 60 minutes, or until a "caramel" starts to ooze out of the pierced holes.

2. Remove the sweet potatoes from the oven, and carefully scoop our their flesh into a large bowl. Add in the milk, flax, nut butter, vanilla, cinnamon, and salt. Use a hand mixer to "cream" the mixture together on for 60 to 90 seconds, starting with the lowest setting. Alternatively, you can place all ingredients into a food processor and blend until thick and smooth, 2 to 3 minutes.

3. Divide into serving bowls, top as desired, and serve warm. Leftovers will keep in the fridge for up to 5 days.

Substitutions: Ground flax can be replaced with ground chia seeds, or omitted.

Tips: If you have large sweet potatoes, I would recommend cutting them in half lengthwise and placing them cut side down on the baking tray to reduce cooking time.

Time Hacks: roasted sweet potatoes are the most sweet and tender, but you can also microwave them for a few minutes in a time crunch. If you already have sweet potato puree and would like to use it in this recipe, use 1 1/3 cups for this recipe (~330 g)

6. Warm Lentil and Tomato Salad

Warm Lentil and Tomato Salad with chilli roasted chickpeas is a delicious vegan meal. Lentils are favourite things to eat, each different type of lentil (red, brown, green, black etc.) carries different qualities, meaning you can fit them in to nearly any meal.

Red lentils are perfect for adding to curries and soups because they break down and become super soft when they're cooked, and the darker colours are perfect for vegan chilli's, burgers, and salads.

The addition of the roasted chickpeas adds a fiery crunchiness, the contrast in texture is what makes this salad super special.

Prep Time: 20 minutes | Cook Time: 30 minutes

Servings: 2

INGREDIENTS

- Lentil Salad/Dressing

- 120 g (1/2 cup) Brown Lentils

- 10-12 Sun Dried Tomatoes

- 2-3 sprigs Fresh Parsley

- 1 tbsp Balsamic Vinegar

- 1 tsp Lemon Juice

- 1 tsp Maple Syrup

- 1 tsp olive oil

- 1/4 tsp Dijon Mustard

- Roasted Chickpeas

- 1 (14oz/400g) Can chickpeas

- 1 tsp olive oil

- 1 tsp Chilli Powder

- 1 pinch Ground Cumin

- 1/4 tsp Ground Turmeric

- 1 pinch Sea Salt

INSTRUCTIONS

1. Preheat the oven to 200°C. Drain and rinse the chickpeas, then dry them as much as possible between two sheets of kitchen paper, removing as much moisture as possible will help them roast nice and crispy.

2. Mix the chickpeas in a bowl with the olive oil and spices until they are evenly coated. Lay them on a flat baking sheet lined with parchment paper and bake for 20 minutes. Allow to cool fully, they will get crispier as they cool as well.

3. While the chickpeas are cooking, bring a saucepan of water to a boil and simmer the lentils for 25-30 minutes, or until completely cooked. While they are cooking whisk together the balsamic vinegar, lemon juice, maple syrup, olive oil and mustard in a separate bowl.

4. Drain the lentils and put back in the saucepan with the dressing. Let the lentils sit in the dressing for 5-10 minutes to absorb some. Slice the sun dried tomatoes and roughly chop the parsley, mix with the lentils.

5. Serve with quinoa and some sliced avocado if you like.

7. Cumin-Roasted Carrot and Golden Beet Soup

This soup is silky in texture, a bit earthy from the beets and cumin.

Ingredients

- 6-7 medium organic carrots, peeled (if desired) and chopped into ½ inch pieces

- 2-3 medium golden beets, peeled (if desired) and chopped into ½ inch cubes (can use red beets but will change the color)

- 2 shallots, chopped into chunks

- 1 Tbsp olive oil (can sub coconut oil or butter/ghee if you do dairy)

- ¼ tsp ground turmeric, divided

- rounded ¼ tsp ground cumin, divided

- ½ tsp dried thyme, divided

- ½ tsp sea salt (I used smoked sea salt for a smoky flavor)

- 2-3 cups bone broth, low-sodium chicken broth or vegetable stock/broth (use veggie if vegan/vegetarian), or more to reach your desired thickness of soup, I prefer a thicker soup

- 2-3 tsp lime juice (or lemon juice for a different flavor)

For serving (optional)

i. chopped cilantro or parsley for serving

ii. Summer squash "cheese" or non-dairy cheese, optional but adds depth of flavor

iii. If you like a little texture in your soup, cubed or sliced avocado

iv. aluminum foil (to create foil packets)

Directions

1. Preheat oven to 400F. Lay two large squares of aluminum foil down, placing carrots in the middle of one square and beets in the middle of the other. Divide the shallots evenly and place on top of each.

2. Combine herbs, spices and salt in a small bowl (turmeric through salt).

3. Drizzle each of the veggies with 1/2 Tbsp of olive oil, then sprinkle the spice mixture evenly over the vegetables.

4. Fold the foil up, creating a seal with each packet and bake for 30 minutes or until tender, the carrots cooked a bit faster than the beets, so check them at 30 minutes.

5. Add roasted veggies and remaining ingredients to a blender and blend until smooth. Top with cilantro or parsley, squash cheese and/or avocado and enjoy warm!

NOTES

If you prefer to roast your carrots and beets on a baking pan instead of in foil packets, that's an option too. I like how the foil packets steam the veggies a bit first and then after opening the pouches, I can brown them a bit.

Stovetop Preparation:

1. You can always sauté the carrots and beets first a bit in a dutch oven, add the spices for 30 seconds until fragrant.

2. Then add broth and remaining ingredients to the pot and bring to a boil. Reduce heat to simmer and let cook until the carrots and beets are tender and soft, about 15-20 minutes.

3. Use an immersion blender to puree or add soup to a blender on high until velvety smooth.

4. Season to taste with more salt and lime juice if desired.

8. Tempeh Kale Taco Salad (Vegan, Gluten-Free)

This festive kale taco salad is packed with a total of over 65g of protein thanks to tempeh and black beans, and irresistible when topped with a creamy cilantro-lime tahini dressing! Lately, If you have been working out more and trying to get more protein into your diet, this salad makes the perfect filling dinner for 2 or 3 servings.

This high-protein vegan taco salad is also great post-workout meal. The kale is soft, after being massaged with lime juice, and corn and cherry. Tomatoes add bright colors and flavors to the salad. You can also top it with creamy avocado and crunchy spiced pepitas.

PREP TIME: 5 MINS | COOK TIME: 10 MINS

Serves: 2-4

Ingredients

- 6 cups kale leaves

- 1 tbsp lime juice

- Tempeh

- 1 8 oz. block tempeh (ensure gluten-free if necessary)

- 2 tbsp tamari

- 1 tbsp lime juice

- ½ tsp onion powder

- ½ tsp cumin

- ¼ tsp chili powder

- 1 tbsp olive oil (optional)

- Cilantro-Lime Tahini

- ¼ cup cilantro leaves

- 3½ tbsp water

- 3 tbsp lime juice

- ½ tsp salt

- 5 level tbsp tahini (sesame paste)

Toppings

- ½ Avocado, sliced

- ⅔ cup corn kernels

- 1 can black beans

- 1½ cup cherry tomatoes, sliced in half

- pepitas

INSTRUCTIONS

1. Massage 1 tbsp lime juice into washed, trimmed kale leaves and place into a salad bowl.

2. Crumble block of tempeh into a medium bowl. Add tamari and lime juice, and stir to coat the tempeh, until it absorbs most of the liquid.

3. Heat olive oil in a medium skillet over medium high heat, and add marinated tempeh.* Add onion powder, cumin, and chili powder. Sauté for about 10 mins, until browned, and remove from heat.

4. Blend all ingredients for cilantro lime tahini in a high speed blender and set aside.

5. Toss kale leaves with tahini dressing, corn, black beans, cherry tomatoes, and crumbled tempeh. Massage the dressing into the kale leaves for best results. Drizzle extra dressing on top, and top with pepitas and sliced avocado if desired. Enjoy!

NOTE

Alternatively, heat 2-4 tbsp water in the skillet and sauté the tempeh until it is softened, adding more water if needed.

9. Zesty Green Soup

This soup has more than one thing going for it — it is easy to make, with simple ingredients, and incorporates lots of goodies you'll want to include. Not to mention it keeps fabulously well in the fridge and freezer. Ginger and garlic are potent additions any time you feel like you are fighting something. Be cautious though — these spices are pretty strong in their raw form, so a little goes a long way.

PREP TIME: 5 MINS | COOK TIME: 25 MINS

Serves: 4

INGREDIENTS

- 2 tbsp solid cooking fat (coconut oil works great here)

- 1 large onion, chopped

- 3 cloves garlic, minced

- 2-in piece ginger, peeled and minced

- 3 cups bone broth

- 1 medium white sweet potato, cubed (about 3 cups)

- 2 small/1 large head of broccoli, chopped (about 1 cup)

- 1 bunch kale, chopped

- 1 lemon, ½ zested and juice reserved

- ½ tsp sea salt

- 1 bunch cilantro

- Avocado for garnish

INSTRUCTIONS

1. Place the fat in the bottom of a heavy-bottomed pot on medium heat. When the fat has melted and the pan is hot, add the onions, and cook, stirring, for 5-7 minutes, or until lightly browned and translucent. Add

the garlic and ginger, and cook for another minute, or until fragrant.

2. Add the bone broth, sweet potato, and broccoli to the pot and bring to a boil. Turn down to a simmer, cover, and cook for 10-15 minutes, or until the vegetables are tender.

3. Turn off the heat, add the kale, half of the bunch of cilantro, lemon zest and juice, and sea salt.

4. Let cool for a few minutes, and blend with a high-powered blender or immersion blender until smooth.

5. Serve warm garnished with avocado and cilantro.

10. Ikarian Taro Root Salad

Taro root, called kolokasi in Greek, is a staplefood on the island of Ikaria and cooked in ways similar to potatoes.

SERVES: 4

Ingredients

- 2 pounds taro root peeled
- Sea salt and freshly ground black pepper
- 1 medium red onion halved and sliced
- 1 small celery stalk chopped
- 1/2 cup chopped fresh parsley
- 8 kalamata olives
- 1/2 cup extra virgin Greek olive oil
- 1 - 2 tablespoons fresh lemon juice

Instructions

1. Scrub the taro under cold running water and peel them with a sharp paring knife, cutting off and discarding the stem ends. Cut the taro into 2-inch / 5-cm cubes.

2. Place in a pot with cold water. Bring to a boil. Reduce heat and simmer until fork tender, about 15 to 20 minutes. Drain and rinse the taro pieces in a colander.

3. Add the onion, celery, parsley, olives, olive oil, and lemon juice. Season to taste with salt and pepper. Toss and serve.

4. The salad may be served either warm or at room temperature.

11. Vegan Turmeric Quinoa Power Bowls

Tumeric is good for everything you cook, especially in quinoa and it tastes amazing. Combine that turmeric quinoa with fresh kale, turmeric roasted potatoes, paprika roasted chickpeas, and a delicious avocado for the most epic Vegan Turmeric Quinoa Power Bowls.

This recipe makes 4 delicious bowls. If you don't have 4 people to feed, they're great for lunch leftovers.

COOK TIME:30 minutes

SERVINGS:4

CALORIES:385 kcal

Ingredients

- 7 small yellow potatoes

- 15 oz. can chickpeas

- 2 tsp turmeric

- 1 tsp paprika

- 1 Tbsp coconut oil

- 1/4 cup quinoa

- salt/pepper

- 2 kale leaves

- 1/2 Tbsp olive oil

- 1 avocado

Instructions

1. Preheat oven to 350 degrees.

2. Slice the potatoes into strips and lay flat on 1/2 of a baking sheet. Spray/drizzle them with coconut oil and sprinkle 1 tsp of turmeric over them. Add salt/pepper to taste.

3. Roast for 5 minutes while you drain and rinse the chickpeas.

4. Place the chickpeas in a mixing bowl and add 1 tsp of paprika, coating them evenly. Lay the chickpeas on the other 1/2 of the baking sheet.

5. Roast the chickpeas and the potatoes for about 25 minutes (or until the potatoes are a little bit soft).

6. Cook the quinoa with 1/2 cup of water. Once the quinoa is cooked, add 1 tsp of turmeric (salt/pepper to taste), mix together, and let cool.

7. Wash the kale and massage the olive oil over the leaves. Separate the leaves into the 4 bowls.

8. Slice the avocado and split into the 4 bowls.

9. Add the quinoa and roasted chickpeas/potatoes to the bowls and serve.

12. Paleo (And Vegan) Zucchini Lasagna with Basil-Cashew Cheese Sauce

This paleo noodleless zucchini lasagna with basil cashew cheese is the right dish for a dairy-free, noodle-less lasagna, this recipe will rock your world.

PREP TIME: 1 hour | COOK TIME: 1 hour 10 mins

Serves: 6-8

INGREDIENTS

- Basil-Cashew Cheese

- 1 cup unsalted cashews

- ½ cup unsweetened almond milk

- ¼ cup fresh basil leaves

- 2 garlic cloves

- ½ teaspoon sea salt

- Artichoke-Tomato Sauce

- 1 tablespoon olive oil

- 1 onion, diced

- 2 garlic cloves, minced

- 14.5-ounce can no-salt-added diced tomatoes

- 8-ounce can no-salt-added tomato sauce

- 1 cup chopped marinated artichoke hearts

- ¼ cup fresh basil leaves, torn into pieces

- Red pepper flakes, to taste

- Sea salt, to taste

- Freshly-ground black pepper, to taste

- Zucchini Lasagna

- 6 medium zucchinis

- Coarse salt

- Fresh basil, for garnish

- Olive oil, for drizzling

INSTRUCTIONS

Basil-Cashew Cheese

1. Soak the cashews in a bowl of water for 30 minutes. Drain and rinse well. Add all the ingredients to a food processor or blender and process/blend until smooth.

Artichoke-Tomato Sauce

2. Heat oil in a medium skillet. Add diced onions and cook for 3-4 minutes, until

onions are softened. Add garlic and cook for 30 minutes, stirring frequently, until fragrant. Next, add the diced tomatoes, tomato sauce, artichoke hearts and basil leaves. Season with red pepper flakes, sea salt and pepper. Bring the sauce to a boil and then simmer on medium low for 10 minutes.

Zucchini Lasagna

3. Preheat oven to 375 degrees F.

4. Slice each zucchini into ⅛-inch thick slices. Salt the zucchini slices heavily and set aside for 20 minutes to drain the water out.

Squeeze as much water out of the zucchini slices as possible.

5. Spread a few tablespoons sauce on the bottom of a casserole dish. Lay 4-5 zucchini slices side-by-side on the bottom of the dish. If you're slices aren't long enough for the entire casserole you can add another vertical row or place some slices horizontally to fill the space.

6. Top the slices with ½ cup sauce and ¼ cup cashew cheese. Repeat with the remaining ingredients, ending with a final layer of sauce and cheese. Garnish with more fresh basil and a drizzle of olive oil.

7. Bake, covered, for 30 minutes and then bake, uncovered for 20-25 minutes or until the top of the lasagna is golden brown. Let the lasagna sit for 15 minutes before cutting and serving. Serve with another drizzle of olive oil.

13. Adrenal Fatigue Recipes: Baked Salmon & Garlic Spinach

This baked salmon and garlic spinach recipe also falls into the paleo category. If you're looking for delicious and easy adrenal fatigue recipes, this baked salmon with garlic spinach is perfect - and so simple to make. The spices you'll use are what bring out the natural flavors of your raw materials.

Prep Time: 5 minutes | Cook Time: 20 minutes

Serves: 2

Ingredients

- 2 salmon filets (5 to 6 ounces each)

- Salt and freshly cracked black pepper to taste

- 6 cups of fresh spinach or 1 lb of frozen spinach

- 3 to 4 large cloves of garlic

- 1/4 tsp + 1/4 tsp of turmeric, divided

- 1/4 tsp of garlic powder

- Couple of squeezes of lemon juice

- 2 tsp + 1 tsp of melted coconut oil, divided

- 1 tbsp. finely chopped parsley

Instructions

1. Preheat oven to 400ºF. Line a baking dish with foil or parchment paper or lightly grease with coconut oil and keep aside.

2. Marinade the salmon with salt and freshly cracked pepper, lemon juice, 1 tsp of melted coconut oil, turmeric, and garlic powder. Arrange a few slices of garlic on the salmon filets (optional). Let it sit while the oven preheats.

3. Once the oven preheats, bake the salmon for about 15 minutes or until it starts flaking.

4. While the salmon is baking, heat the coconut oil in a pan and fry the garlic for about 30 seconds to 1 minute. Add the spinach and cook until the spinach wilts.

5. If you are using frozen spinach, there will be extra liquid. Cook till the water evaporates or pour off. Season with freshly cracked black pepper and salt.

6. Plate and serve your salmon spinach recipe.

7. Serve the baked salmon on a bed of cooked garlicky spinach.

14. Bolognese Sauce with Chicken Livers and Zoodles

Organ meats are the most concentrated source of just about every nutrient, including important vitamins, minerals, healthy fats and essential amino acids.

Servings: serves 4-6

Ingredients

- 2 tbsp solid fat, divided
- 1 large onion, finely chopped
- 2 large carrots, chopped
- 1 large beetroot, grated
- 2 sticks celery, chopped
- 310g pastured chicken livers, chopped

- 900g grass fed beef

- 3 cups (500ml) beef stock

- 3 tbsp coconut aminos

- 2 bay leaves

- 6 stems fresh thyme

- 1 Tbsp fresh rosemary, chopped

- 1 tsp salt

Instructions

1. Preheat the oven to 250°F/130°C.

2. Heat 1 tbsp fat in a large lidded casserole (Dutch oven), add the onion and sauté on a low heat for approx 8-10 minutes until softened and translucent. Add the celery, carrots and beetroot to the pan and cook a

further 5 minutes, then remove everything to a plate and set to one side.

3. Put the other tablespoon fat into the pan, add the livers and cook 2 minutes on a medium heat. Add the beef and cook for another 5 minutes. Add the reserved vegetables, together with the herbs, stock and coconut aminos. Bring to the boil, cover with the lid and place in the oven.

4. Cook for as long as you possibly can, but for a minimum of 3 hours, checking a couple of times to make sure the sauce is not drying up. I will happily let mine sit in the oven for 5-6 hours, the longer the better, I think, to let all those flavours develop nicely. When it

looks and tastes rich and satisfying, you're good to go.

5. Remove the bay leaves and leafless thyme stems and serve over courgette 'noodles' (zoodles).

Zoodles

- 4 large courgettes (zucchini)
- 1 tbsp solid fat

Instructions

1. Cut the ends off each courgette and peel the skin if you wish.

2. Using a spiraliser or a julienne peeler, make long 'noodles' from each courgette. Heat the

fat in a large sauté pan, then add the courgette.

3. Cook for about 5 minutes until tender, or however you like to serve them, being careful not to overcook them or they will break up.

15. Anti-Inflammatory Smoothie

This Anti-Inflammatory Smoothie contains ginger, beets and greens to help reduce inflammation in your body. This recipe is plant based and help you fuel your body so you can go after your passions, it is good for dessert or food replacement smoothie.

Over the last few years, many studies have shown that inflammation contributes to a number of health conditions and symptoms. Things like skin rashes, digestive troubles, headaches and migraines, brain fog, fatigue, and more can often be attributed to inflammation.

FOODS THAT CAUSE INFLAMMATION

The foods that cause inflammation won't surprise you. Red meat, processed and preserved meats and sausage, dairy, gluten and white flours/starches, refined sugar, and preservatives top the list. A diet rich in these potent foods will most likely cause you to feel cruddy anyway. If you're susceptible to inflammation, these things can make symptoms even worse.

Focus on foods that are very similar to a Mediterranean diet, making it super doable for most people in the western world. Here's the list to focus on:

- tomatoes
- olive oil
- leafy greens + cruciferous veggies
- fruit, berries + other low glycemic fruits
- citrus – lemons and oranges
- fish rich in omega-3 fatty acids – salmon, sardines, mackerel
- ginger

- garlic

- turmeric

ANTI-INFLAMMATORY RECIPES

Green smoothies can help tremendously if you're struggling to add anti-inflammatory foods to your diet. I combine quite a few of the ingredients listed above into this smoothie recipe. It's nutrient-packed and makes the perfect anti-inflammatory smoothie.

Prep Time: 10 minutes | Yield: 2 servings

Ingredients

- 1 cup baby kale

- 1/2 small beet (peeled and chopped)

- 1/2 cup water

- 1/2 orange (peeled)

- 1 cup mixed berries (frozen)

- 1/2 cup pineapple (frozen)

- 1 tsp fresh ginger (grated or chopped)

- 1 tsp coconut oil

Instructions

1. Place baby kale, beet, water, and orange into a blender.

2. Puree until smooth.

3. Add remaining ingredients.

4. Blend again until smooth.

Notes

i. Carrots can be substituted for the beets.

ii. Mango can be substituted for the pineapple.

16. Adrenal Fatigue Green Smoothie

This Adrenal Fatigue Green Smoothie is chock full of nutritious ingredients chosen for their anti-inflammatory and adrenal-supporting properties. Baby spinach is high in iron and contains moderate amounts of vitamins B6 and C. Cauliflower is high in vitamin C, and is a great source of B6, and magnesium.

Coconut water provides extra B6, magnesium, and iron. Pineapple is extremely high in vitamin C, and one cup provides another 10% RDV of B-6 and 5% magnesium. Turmeric is well-known for its anti-inflammatory properties thanks to curcumin, but it's also high in iron and B6. Finally flax oil is one of the best sources of omega-3 fatty acids. This smoothie is hydrating and full of heart- and GI-tract-friendly dietary fiber.

MUSHROOM ELIXIR FOR ADRENAL FATIGUE

Another helpful way to combat adrenal fatigue is to include adaptogenic herbs in your diet. They can better help your body respond to stress and recharge the adrenal glands.

The best adaptogens for stress are rhodiola, mucuna pruriens, ashwaganda, cordyceps, schisandra, and licorice root. Maca and ginseng are great for fatigue.

But a word of caution, discuss using these herbs with your healthcare provider as some adaptogens may interact with any prescription medications or supplements.

This smoothie contains specially chosen ingredients to help the adrenal glands recover and support health and wellness.

Prep Time: 5 minutes | Yield: 1 smoothie

Ingredients

- 1 cup baby spinach (fresh)

- 1/2 cup coconut water (unsweetened)

- 1/2 orange (peeled)

- 1 cup pineapple (cubed, fresh or frozen)

- 1/2 cup cauliflower florets (frozen)

- 1 tablespoon fresh turmeric (or 1 teaspoon ground turmeric)

- 1 tablespoon flax oil

Instructions

1. Place spinach, coconut water, and orange in blender.

2. Puree until smooth.

3. Add pineapple, cauliflower, turmeric, flax oil, and any adaptogenic herbs, if using.

4. Blend again.

Notes

If using adaptogenic herbs, use according to package directions for specific type and always check with a medical professional before using as some may cause interactions with prescription medications.

17. Adrenals Half Full Signature Mocktail

Adrenals Half Full Signature Mocktail is the perfect drink to add to your daily routine as a way to support your adrenal glands. If your adrenals need a little reboot and extra adrenal support after a crazy busy holiday season, this Adrenals Half Full Signature Mocktail is the perfect drink to add to your daily routine as a way to support your adrenal glands. Plus it's delicious and easy to make.

Our mocktail is made with holy basil (tulsi leaf) tea, sparkling mineral water, Himalayan sea salt, fresh organic oranges, fresh basil, and a touch of grade B maple syrup for those who like it a tad on the sweet side.

How the Adrenals Half Full Signature Mocktail for Adrenal Support works:

Holy basil is an adaptogenic herb that supports the adrenal glands. Adaptogens help the adrenals, you guessed it, "adapt" the way they react to stressors by supporting a more balanced hormonal response.

Sparkling mineral water helps hydrate the body, and also contains essential minerals.

Himalayan sea salt contains trace minerals, which are important when it comes to supporting the adrenals. Those suffering with adrenal fatigue often find their body has a hard time regulating sodium due to the reduction of the hormone aldosterone.

Oranges are a great source of Vitamin C & bioflavonoids. These all-star micronutrients assist the body in hormone production, and protecting it against free radical damage by virtue of their antioxidant ability.

Grade B maple syrup is an alkaline forming sweetener that is not only delicious, but also contains essential minerals and B-vitamins that are necessary for energy production and adrenal hormone production.

Prep Time: 15 min | **Cook Time**: 5 min

Yield: 2

Ingredients

- 2 bags of Tulsi Tea (holy basil)
- 16 oz of filtered water
- 1/4 teaspoon pink Himalayan sea salt
- 2 oranges (freshly squeezed)
- 1/2–1 Tablespoon grade B maple syrup (optional)
- 16 oz of sparkling mineral water

- Fresh basil leaves to taste (we recommend thinly slicing 2 basil leaves)

Instructions

1. Heat filtered water on the stove top, removing from heat prior to water boiling. Ideal temperature would be 208-212° F. Let steep in Tulsi Tea bags for 4 minutes.

2. Remove tea bags and place in freezer to cool.

3. Add Himalayan sea salt, the juice of 2 oranges, grade B maple syrup (optional) and whisk to combine. Store overnight in an airtight container or mason jar.

4. Prior to drinking, add 16 ounces sparkling mineral water and fresh sliced basil leaves, and stir to combine.

18. Cinnamon Spice Kombucha

A fermented tea, kombucha is a lively, fizzy probiotic beverage that is at once faintly tart with hints of apple cider. In this version, classic kombucha tea undergoes a second fermentation that infuses it with the flavors of cinnamon, cloves, ginger and sweet spices.

What is kombucha?

Kombucha is a traditionally fermented tea that, like all fermented foods, is extraordinarily rich in beneficial bacteria – those same bacteria that help to support gut health and immune system function.   And, like most fermented foods, kombucha is blessedly simple to make – requiring little more effort or knowledge than you'd need in making a simple sweet tea. Kombucha is brewed and fermented by the way of a SCOBY, or a symbiotic colony of bacteria and yeasts.

How to Brew Kombucha

Kombucha tea is now widely available in health food stores and in many supermarkets where it is priced at about $3 to $5 for a bottle. Fortunately, making kombucha is easy – involving little more than heating water, steeping tea and sweetening it before pouring it into a vessel with a kombucha mother to ferment. The kombucha mother performs the bulk of the work as beneficial bacteria and yeasts consume the sugar in the sweet tea, and transform it into a wonderfully tart, probiotic-rich kombucha tea.

Secondary fermentation of kombucha also allows the opportunity to flavor your kombucha by adding fruit juices, herbs or spices. In my favorite wintertime version of kombucha, I flavor it with sweet spices and a touch of sweet apple cider that provides enough carbohydrate to give the kombucha fuel for its much-needed fizz.

Servings: 1 quart

Ingredients

- 2 whole cloves

- 1 ceylon cinnamon stick about 3 inches long

- 1 teaspoon grated ginger

- 3 tablespoons apple juice

- 1 ¾ cup kombucha tea

Instructions

1. Drop the cloves and cinnamon stick into a 16-ounce flip-top bottle.

2. In a pitcher, stir the grated ginger and apple juice into the kombucha tea. Pour the liquid ingredients into the flip-top bottle, leaving at least ½ inch of headspace. Close the bottle,

and transfer it to a warm spot in your kitchen.

3. Allow the kombucha to ferment for 5 days, then transfer to the refrigerator.

4. Open the bottle carefully over the sink as it may foam, and strain the kombucha through a fine mesh sieve.

5. Serve the kombucha over ice.

Recipe Notes

To prepare this recipe for Cinnamon Spice Kombucha, you must first have brewed kombucha tea which is then mixed with sweet apple cider and spices to produce a flavored, fizzy drink.

19. Adrenal Recovery Soup

Make this delicious recovery soup recipe for a healthy recovery from fatigue. A 100% healthy choice to assist with recovery. A vegetable soup proved helpful in restoring adrenal function. Plus it's low-cal, packed with vitamins and healthy.

Servings: 4

Ingredients

- 2 Courgette (finely chopped)
- 2 Onions (finely chopped)
- 200 g Green beans
- 3 Cloves garlic
- 8 Ripe Tomatoes (chopped)
- 5 Celery stocks

- Tbsp Fresh Coriander

- 600 ml Vegetable stock

- 2 Tsp Smoked paprika

- 1 Tbsp olive oil

- Salt & Pepper

Instructions

1. Sauté your onion, garlic, coriander & olive oil Add in your courgette, celery, smoked paprika, green beans and sauté for 10mins.

2. Add in your chopped tomatoes and your vegetable stock (We recommend using the Kallo yeast, gluten and lactose-free stock cube, also free from MSG).

3. Bring to the boil and simmer for 20mins

20. Sourdough Rye Crepes with Sorghum-Cinnamon Apples

Ingredients

For the Crepes

- 3 eggs

- 1 ½ cups sourdough starter

- ¼ teaspoon finely ground real salt

- ¼ cup whole milk

- 3 tablespoons butter plus extra for the pan

- 1 tablespoon sorghum molasses available here

- ½ teaspoon ground ceylon cinnamon

For the Apples

- ¼ cup butter

- 2 large apples cored and sliced thin

- 2 tablespoons of sorghum molasses

- Pinch finely ground real salt

- ½ teaspoon ground ceylon cinnamon

Instructions

1. Place a 10" cast-iron skillet over medium heat.

2. In a medium-sized mixing bowl, whisk the eggs. Add the sourdough starter, sea salt,

milk, melted butter, sorghum molasses, and cinnamon and whisk well to combine.

3. Once the cast-iron skillet is pre-heated, add a teaspoon of butter and allow to melt. Quickly pour half of a soup ladle full of crepe batter into the pan in a swirled circle pattern, starting in the center of the pan. Grab the skillet handle with a gloved hand or hotpad and tilt the pan in a circular motion, allowing the batter to form a thin, circle on the bottom of the pan.

4. Allow to cook 3-4 minutes, or until the edges are completely dry and the center is firm, and carefully slide a spatula beneath the crepe. Carefully flip and allow to cook 3

more minutes. Move cooked crepes to a waiting plate.

5. Continue cooking remaining crepes, adding a teaspoon of cooking fat before each one.

6. Once all of the crepes are cooked, add 4 Tablespoons of butter to the pan and allow to melt before adding the sliced apples. Cook for several minutes, stirring occasionally.

7. Spoon in the sorghum molasses and sprinkle over the salt and cinnamon. Stir and cook for 3-5 minutes, or until the apples are just starting to soften and the butter-sorghum mixture has coated the apples in a caramel-like sauce.

8. To serve, layout two crepes per person and divide the apples amongst the plates. Roll up and drizzle the syrup in the pan over the crepes.

Recipe Notes

Considering that the recipe requires no additional flour, the grains are fully fermented and don't weigh us down after a meal, when we need that energy for keeping up with the chickens or the children.

Sorghum Molasses

A perfect compliment to the rye and apples is sorghum molasses, a sweetener that comes not from sugar cane as we are familiar with, but a variety of "sweet sorghum" which is cousin to grain sorghum. It is made by cooking the juice from the stalk of the Sorghum plant into a sweet, thick syrup. Somewhere in flavor between molasses and honey, it contains nutrients such as iron, calcium, and potassium.

And combined with butter and apples, it makes a caramel apple-like filling for these delicious and simple crepes.

Sorghum molasses can be found all across the southern United States, as well as in many health food stores.

Tangy sourdough rye crepes filled with fall apples and lightly sweetened with sorghum molasses makes a comforting fall dessert or breakfast. As breakfast it is recommended to serve it alongside bacon or eggs and cinnamon-spiked milk kefir.

21. Sprouted Spelt Crepes

Using sprouted spelt flour as in this recipe – or even sprouted soft white wheat provides a boost of fiber and micronutrients to the dish. We serve these with fruit and a cultured dairy food like kefir, yogurt or viili. As a tasty alternative to sweet crepes, serve them with lox, steamed asparagus and hollandaise sauce. Sprouted grain is rich in nutrients and enjoys an increased level of vitamins than its non-sprouted counterparts.

Servings: 14 – 15 crepes

Ingredients

- 2 eggs

- 1 ¼ Cup whole milk

- 1 Cup Organic Sprouted Spelt our Sprouted White Wheat Flour

- Pinch finely ground real salt

- butter

Instructions

1. Mix all ingredients except butter or coconut oil together until thoroughly blended. Eliminate all lumps of flour.

2. Set the batter aside for 1 to 2 hours. This gives you the opportunity to prep other dishes you might serve.

3. Heat a tablespoon or so of butter or coconut oil in a skillet or crepe pan over medium heat until melted.

4. Pour 2 to 3 tablespoons of batter into the heated pan and swirl the batter around the pan quickly so as to distribute the batter thinly.

5. Cook the crepe for 30 to 45 seconds or until small bubbles begin to appear in the batter, flip the crepe and cook the other side for 30 seconds.

6. Remove from the pan to a warm plate.

7. Continue this process until all your batter has been exhausted and adding butter or coconut oil to the pan as needed. Don't worry if you lose a few of those first crepes while you perfect your technique.

22. Homemade Yogurt & Spelt Crackers

Homemade crackers are well-loved in our home – rustic, flavorful and tender, they've become a favorite of both visiting children and adults. In our version of homemade crackers, we rely on whole grain flour for its rich and earthy flavor and nutritive value. First whole grain flour is combined with fresh yogurt, and allowed to rest overnight which fulfills the dual purpose of not only improve the tenderness of the grain, but also improving its nutrient profile.

All whole grains contain antinutrients – naturally present substances like food phytates which keep the grain from sprouting until conditions for the plants growth are optimal, but also bind up with minerals in our digestive tracts, preventing their full absorption.

In this recipe for homemade crackers, we use whole, full-fat yogurt to soak the flour before combining the dough with good quality grass-fed butter, which creates a flaky texture and crumb. Season the crackers with coarse sea salt, dried chives or dill, or leave them plain, anyway you make them is worth your time and effort. Consider adding dried herbs to the dough for a variation in flavor.

Prep Time: 20 mins | Cook Time: 7 mins

Servings: 120 crackers (12 Servings)

Ingredients

- 3 cups spelt flour buy spelt flour here

- 1 teaspoon finely ground real salt I use this one

- 1 cup yogurt try making raw milk yogurt

- ½ cup butter plus 2 tablespoons melted butter

Instructions

1. Stir three cups whole grain spelt flour and one teaspoon unrefined sea salt with one cup full fat yogurt in the bowl of a stand mixer equipped with a dough hook. Continue to process until the dough forms a smooth ball.

2. Place the dough in a mixing bowl and cover it with a tea cloth. Leave the dough to rest at room temperature overnight and up to twenty-four hours.

3. Once the dough has rested overnight or up to a full day, preheat the oven to 450 degrees Fahrenheit.

4. Knead one-half cup softened butter into the dough, then divide the it into four separate balls to make rolling it more manageable.

5. Flour your working surface and your rolling pin, place one ball of dough into the center of your work surface and roll it to ⅛-inch. Cut the dough into rounds with a biscuit cutter, or into triangles or squares with a pizza cutter or sharp knife.

6. Brush each unbaked cracker with melted butter, prick with the tines of a fork to prevent puffing and bake in an oven preheated to 450 degrees Fahrenheit until brown and crispy, about six or seven minutes.

23. Homemade Yogurt

Homemade yogurt is a staple in our home. Easy to prepare, inexpensive, delicious and nourishing, we manage to go through about a half-gallon of fresh, homemade yogurt each week. A probiotic food, homemade yogurt contains live beneficial bacteria that help to colonize the gut with microbiota that are essential to the proper functioning of your immune system, digestion and the ability of your body to manufacture critical nutrients.

In addition to a wealth of beneficial bacteria, homemade yogurt is also rich in other nutrients. The process of lactic acid fermentation allows beneficial bacteria to metabolize lactose – a sugar naturally present in milk.   The end result of this process results in a dairy product that is lower in carbohydrates and higher in b vitamins including folic acid than regular whole milk.   Furthermore, many people who find they're intolerant or sensitive to lactose find that they can eat yogurt and other cultured dairy foods without much reaction. Reduced lactose content coupled with the solidity of the milk product may both contribute to increased digestibility of yogurt and other cultured dairy foods.

Thermophilic Homemade Yogurt & Mesophilic Homemade Yogurt

Homemade yogurt can be either thermophilic or mesophilic. That is, homemade yogurt is cultured either in a warm, heated environment (thermophilic) or a room temperature environment (mesophilic). The yogurts you're accustomed to eating are usually thermophilic yogurts; however, room temperature yogurt presents an easy-to-prepare alternative with many variations in texture and flavor. For instance, piima is a homemade Scandinavian yogurt with a runny texture and almost cheesy flavor while viili, another homemade yogurt cultured at room temperature, is mildly sweet and gelatinous.

Prep Time: 10 mins | Fermentation: 6 hrs

Servings: 4 servings (1 quart)

Ingredients

- 4 cups whole milk

- ¼ cup yogurt starter

Instructions

1. Bring the milk to a simmer over medium-high heat. When it reaches 180 F, turn off the heat and allow the milk to cool to 110 F.

2. Whisk the yogurt starter into the warm milk, and pour it into a quart-sized jar. Set the milk into a yogurt maker, and allow it to culture at least 6 and up to 12 hours. The longer it cultures, the sourer it will taste.

3. Transfer the yogurt to the fridge and use within a month.

FINAL THOUGHT

The adrenal fatigue diet has been successful in increasing energy levels and regulating blood pressure because it promotes healthier eating habits and lifestyle changes.

This diet also doesn't require any major dietary restrictions that could harm your health. However, you should talk with your doctor before changing eating habits.

If you begin to experience any adverse symptoms or if the diet makes your condition worse, visit your doctor immediately.

The adrenal fatigue diet is still being tested. This is partly because doctors are still researching adrenal fatigue. But, it's been proven that eating a healthier diet and adopting a healthier lifestyle can make you feel better physically and mentally.